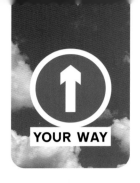

'Your Way' summarizes the ideas found in the booklet. Managing your diabetes is all about finding out what works for you on an individual level; experimenting with different levels of exercise, insulin and food intake; taking control of and responsibility for your diabetes; listening to your body and operating within its limits.

Finding out how to do this is hard, though, and the purpose of Joe's Rough Guide to Diabetes is to help you achieve it.

Handily, 'YOUR WAY' also forms a neat acronym of the seven points you need to remember to achieve a good basic level of control!

You're responsible
for your diabetes

Only you
can work out how to control your diabetes

Urgent assistance
is required if you have ketoacidosis

Remember to measure
your glucose level before and after you do something new

Whenever you travel
take extra supplies

Always carry
something sweet on you

You have a hidden disability,
but don't let it stop you living your life

Designed and typeset in 10pt Trade Gothic by Gary Brown, for Joe's Diabetes Ltd, London, UK

Printed and bound by Regal Litho Ltd, Unit 3, Enigma Building, Bilton Road,
Denbigh East, MK1 1HW

ISBN 978-0-9564117-0-9

CONTENTS

FOREWORD TO THE FIRST EDITION

Becoming diabetic at any age means a complete change in lifestyle, but for those in their teens and early 20s the challenges of diabetes are completely at odds with what is supposed to be happening in their lives. At a time of rapid growth, when raiding fridges and consuming junk food is the norm, they have to be careful about what they eat and drink. They are supposed to be developing independence and experimenting with life but their friends and families keep checking on them. So it should come as no surprise to discover that measures of diabetes control are at their worst during these difficult times. How difficult is it to be just like your peers when you're doing blood tests and having injections? So what can be done to help?

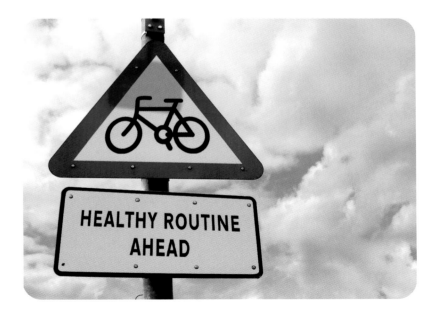

Knowing a lot about diabetes is not the same as knowing how to live with diabetes and this is where Joseph's booklet is so very different from the usual guides. Not only does he give an excellent factual account of diabetes, he also shares his experiences of solving many related problems. And it is not just the obvious things such as dealing with high or low blood sugars that Joseph covers; he also tackles issues such as drug and alcohol use that many health professionals find awkward to deal with.

I have learnt that the only thing young people with diabetes share is a need to inject insulin. They each develop their own strategies to manage their diabetes but at the same time find it helpful to share experiences with other diabetic peers, though that can be very difficult to arrange. This booklet offers such an opportunity, with a host of practical ideas developed by somebody living with diabetes. It ought to be available to every young diabetic and be essential reading to anybody involved in helping young people to grow up with diabetes.

Dr Bill Lamb MD FRCP FRCPCH
Consultant Paediatrician
Bishop Auckland Hospital
County Durham

FOREWORD TO THE SECOND EDITION

Joe's Rough Guide to Diabetes is a brilliant presentation of a journey in a diabetic patient's life, which combines some established rules with the practicalities of everyday life.

It is right to say that a Type 1 diabetic individual is their "own best doctor". This reflects the fact that although Type 1 diabetes is characterised by an established process with loss of endogenous insulin production, its control presents different challenges to each patient.

Joe's guide embraces the concept "I am my own best doctor" and offers practical instructions and advice, mostly derived from the direct experience of an individual living with diabetes who has learnt to know himself.

The book is spontaneous, authoritative, and most importantly real. It would certainly help any young patient to promote that sense of responsibility and perhaps curiosity that should drive every Type 1 diabetic to pursue good metabolic control.

Dr Luigi Gnudi MD PhD FRCP FASN

Reader in Diabetes and Metabolic Medicine
Honorary Consultant in Diabetes and Endocrinology
King's College London

1. INTRODUCTION

This booklet is simply a guide to living with diabetes, not a definitive medical document. I was diagnosed with Type 1 diabetes when I was 13 years old. Whilst there were very good pieces of literature concerning diabetes from the NHS, none of them ever seemed to make an attempt to give real-life examples. Consequently, I had to learn for myself, mainly by trial and error. This prompted me to write this booklet, to advise others in a similar position, to the best of my understanding, how to live and enjoy life as much as possible without a fully functioning pancreas! Hopefully, the ten years of experience I have can go to help others who find themselves in the position I was in, when I was diagnosed. I hope that this guide will help you avoid some of the bumps and pitfalls which I encountered.

One of the distinctive features of Type 1 diabetes is that it is self-medicated. This means that in the day-to-day running of things you are effectively your own doctor. This is not to say that you should ignore your own healthcare professionals, far from it, but all they can do is advise from a distance, whereas you should know what to do, and what is happening in a diabetic sense, from moment to moment.

> **When you have diabetes you are effectively your own doctor! You should know what to do, and what is happening, from moment to moment.**

Having said that please remember I am not a doctor, just a person with first-hand experience of controlling my diabetes. I am telling you what works for me, which you can adapt to your own circumstances.

Please remember you should discuss any problems about your own condition with your own healthcare team.

The only way to achieve perfect control is to think of your body as a machine. Calculating how much insulin you require can make the difference between you having a good and a bad day, so it is best to be exact. The more exact you are, the more in control you are, and the healthier and happier you should be.

The constant thinking, measuring and injecting can be very tiring, and even depressing, if you cannot achieve control.

It is also important to remember that being diabetic should not over-ride your life as this would definitely lead to unhappiness! However, awareness of your diabetes should always be in your sub-conscious. This is the tedious thing about it – the repetition. The repetition of thought, the painful measuring and the repetition of injecting on a daily basis can be very tiring and quite possibly depressing if you cannot achieve control. If this occurs, contact your healthcare team or diabetic nurse and they should be able to help.

Here's the rub though: you are only human. Mistakes will happen, despite your best intentions, and the wishes of the team. It is this humanity that complicates diabetic control, and yet it is for being human and enjoying life that you control your blood glucose level. Effectively, being a good diabetic means continuous thought before any action is taken. What to think is another matter – and this is where this guide should come in handy. I hope it helps and that I have not rambled on too much.

2. SO... YOU HAVE TYPE 1 DIABETES

Being diabetic isn't easy and being told you have diabetes is even harder. It's not that it is such a terrible disease, in comparison with cancer for example, but it does force a change in how you live your life that in some senses curtails your freedom. People react to this loss of freedom in different ways depending on age, maturity and how they lived their lives before being diagnosed. Personally, I found it very difficult to cope psychologically. The first year was particularly difficult, hampered as I was by, possibly psychosomatically-induced, chronic sinusitis, which meant I missed out on most of that school year and the developing social life associated with it. This made life doubly depressing since whilst I felt horrible most of the time and didn't want to see anyone, the feeling that I was being left behind in a social sense was tangible. If you have problems of a similar nature or cannot come to terms with being diagnosed – and it is a large shock – do contact your healthcare team and you should be able to get some counselling.

GO

It can often be hard to express your feelings. especially about coming to terms with your diagnosis — but it is always best to try.

Often it can be hard to express these feelings but it is always best to try. Alternatively, some people find that writing, painting or exercise (see Chapter 4) can help when counselling cannot. If one doesn't work, don't get depressed and think that nothing can help; give it a chance and then give it up if it doesn't help and try something new. I know the following statement doesn't help in the short term, but life does get better and easier the longer you have the disease since you should gain more control over it. Having said this, it seems to take people 'on average' about two years or more to really adjust to being diagnosed. The first year is taken up with shock and learning to accommodate the disease into your life. In the second year you realise that the disease is not going to go away, even if you control it well. Coping with this problem is not something I can help with, but I can help you control your disease.

What is the problem? The Biology of Diabetes

You've probably already been told this by your team but with diabetes repetition is the key!

Type 1 diabetes is due to damage to the Islets of Langerhans in the pancreas. These are clusters of hormone-secreting cells scattered throughout the pancreas.

Fig.1 The location of the pancreas

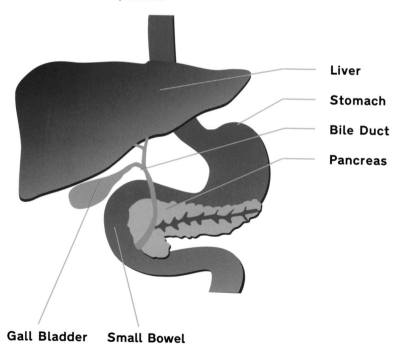

Liver

Stomach

Bile Duct

Pancreas

Gall Bladder   Small Bowel

The damage can be caused by a variety of factors: some babies are born with diabetes, other children develop it a few years later. My own diabetes is thought to have developed after a viral infection. No matter how you get it, diabetes is caused by an autoimmune response; that is, the body's immune system gets confused and attacks the beta cells of the Islets of Langerhans. These cells produce insulin, which is a hormone (a chemical messenger in the blood). The insulin controls the amount of glucose (sugar) in the blood by telling the cells how much glucose they should allow in.

Fig.2 Blood glucose and hormone release

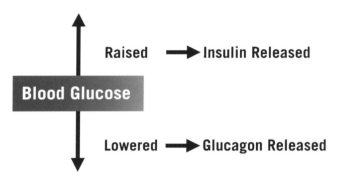

Typically when a person eats, food is absorbed into the blood and the body releases insulin to lower the blood glucose level. The glucose goes into tissues such as the muscles, brain and kidneys to provide energy, and excess glucose goes into fat and is stored. If the blood glucose level is too low, the body releases a different hormone called glucagon, which raises the blood glucose level by slowing down insulin production and breaking down the body's medium-term energy store (glycogen) into glucose, the sugar in the blood. Glycogen is found mainly in the liver and muscles.

By this method the body keeps the blood glucose level constant at around 5 mmol/L of glucose per litre of blood, (mmol is a millimole

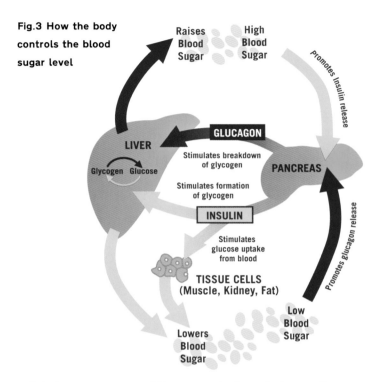

Fig.3 How the body controls the blood sugar level

Raises Blood Sugar — High Blood Sugar

Promotes insulin release

GLUCAGON

LIVER

Glycogen Glucose

Stimulates breakdown of glycogen

Stimulates formation of glycogen

PANCREAS

INSULIN

Stimulates glucose uptake from blood

TISSUE CELLS (Muscle, Kidney, Fat)

Promotes glucagon release

Lowers Blood Sugar — Low Blood Sugar

– it is just a measure of the amount of a substance. If you are doing chemistry at school you will learn more about millimoles.)

People with Type 1 diabetes do not have the luxury of this 'automatic' system. Since no insulin is produced naturally by the body when we eat, we have to inject insulin. However, this leads to complications. To keep the blood glucose level constant we need to take precisely the right amount. This is very far from easy to calculate (see p.55). If too much is taken then the blood glucose level will fall. Glucagon is released but its effect in raising the blood glucose is quite slow, since the body does not react in the same way to injected insulin as it does to its own 'home-grown' variety. This leads to hypoglycaemia, where there is not enough glucose in the blood.

Hypoglycaemia

The classic response to a 'hypo' is a release of glucagon and an adrenalin surge as the body attempts to raise the blood glucose level (adrenalin raises blood glucose). The symptoms of an adrenalin rush are shaking, a pale face, cold hands, a faster breathing rate, and an increased heart rate. As there is not enough glucose for the brain to function properly, the person may also have slurred speech, double vision, seizures, feel very hungry and in the later stages be confused. They may also undergo personality changes, possibly expressing anger or aggression. Not everyone will have all of these symptoms.

If left untreated, hypoglycaemia can lead to a diabetic coma.

Symptoms of hypoglycaemia
- Shaking
- Pale face
- Cold hands
- Faster breathing rate
- Increased heart rate
- Slurred speech
- Double vision
- Seizures
- Hunger
- Confusion
- Anger
- Aggression

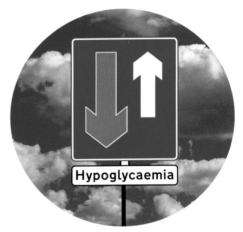

A typical reading on a blood glucose measuring machine for a 'hypo' feeling can be anywhere below 5mmol/L but between 3mmol/L and 1 mmol/L is more common. Readings below 3mmol/L require immediate action! See Chapter 3 for how to manage a 'hypo'.

Hyperglycaemia

This is exactly the opposite of hypoglycaemia; it occurs when not enough insulin has been injected for the amount of food eaten, so there is too much glucose in the blood. A typical reading on a glucose meter for hyperglycaemia is above 10 mmol/L. Symptoms include feeling tired and 'groggy', making concentration difficult. People with hyperglycaemia will feel thirsty and pee a lot more often as the body tries to expel as much glucose as possible (the thirst is a direct result of this loss of fluid). If left untreated not much will happen in the short term, apart from you not feeling too good and possibly having a thrush infection in your mouth or genitals.

Symptoms of hyperglycaemia
- Tiredness
- Feeling 'groggy'
- Difficulty concentrating
- Thirst
- Urinating a lot

However, years of poor control of your diabetes and long-term hyperglycaemia can lead to blindness (diabetic retinopathy), the loss of feeling in your hands and feet (neuropathy), and death from heart disease. This is because the inner lining of the blood vessels becomes stickier and the blood flow is reduced, making the vessels more likely to clog. In men this can also cause impotence. (There you have it guys, don't let it get up or you won't be able to get it up any more!)

Long term consequences of poor diabetic control
- Blindness
- Loss of sensation in feet and hands
- Ulceration of feet
- Heart disease
- Kidney disease
- Impotence

Treatment for hyperglycaemia includes exercise (see Chapter 4), but only when there is some insulin in the system (long-acting insulin counts) and/or possibly an extra insulin injection, preferably of just fast-acting insulin. If your blood glucose rises to 15 mmol/L or more and you feel poorly you should take action. If no insulin is taken ketoacidosis can occur, which is life-threatening. See how to treat hyperglycaemia and avoid ketoacidosis in Chapter 3.

3. DAY-TO-DAY LIVING

So you've come over the first hurdle of actually being told you have diabetes and realising your life is going to change drastically. Now comes the next one which is the key to control – the Routine and what happens when your control is not so good! Most people who have diabetes, and lots of those who don't, have heard about 'hypos' and diabetic comas.

People who are hypoglycaemic may often be taken as drunk; identification can avoid this confusion.

STOP

CARRY I.D

How to handle hypoglycaemia and hyperglycaemia

Hypoglycaemia, as we saw in Chapter 2, is very low blood glucose, which can lead to a coma. The treatment then is basically anything sweet you can lay your hands on. I am told the preferred option of the medical establishment is a sweet fizzy drink and specifically Lucozade™ or dextrose tablets. However, anything sweet will do, but remember not all sugars are absorbed as fast as glucose, and liquids are absorbed more quickly than solids. A spoonful of sugar isn't actually absorbed that quickly; you are much better taking glucose, or corn sugar.

So make sure that you always carry something sweet about your person. This can be anything from a GlucoGel© (formerly known as Hypostop™) to dextrose tablets to mints or chocolate bars, but it is very important to "be prepared" (to steal a famous phrase). An alternative to glucose sweets (that taste horrible) are things like Starbursts®. This advice applies 24 hours a day since your insulin doesn't stop working just because you're asleep. Going hypo in your sleep is a worry, but you should be OK: unless you've lost your feeling or are heavily drugged, the adrenalin should wake you up. It tends to ruin your rest for the night as, though you'll go back to sleep, you won't wake up refreshed. Anyway, keep some food near your bed as it's bad enough waking up with your heart racing without having to stumble down to the kitchen to sort it out.

Control can never be perfect, even in day-to-day living, and if you are undertaking a new regime or activity it is essential to have a 'safety net' to fall back on. There are not many things more worrying than to think that you're going hypo with no means of saving yourself. Personally, I always carry around with me a GlucoGel© at least, and I usually have some chocolate bars secreted away in a coat or jacket.

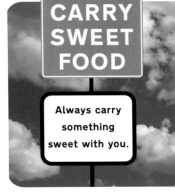

Also you should wear, or have in your wallet or purse, some form of identity that shows you are diabetic. Several companies produce tags and bracelets; you can search on the Diabetes UK website or on the internet. This is crucial, especially if you are drinking alcohol (see Chapter 5) since you may be too drunk to realise you're hypo, and by the time someone does, it may be too late and you're in a coma. Ideally, you should also have someone with you who knows what to look out for if you are in trouble. However, this person should also know that it is not their job to 'nanny' you and ask if you are OK all the time; not many things could be more annoying.

As a side note, it is worth remembering to measure every time you think you're hypo. There have been a number of times when I've been tired and hungry and just eaten because I felt hypo-ish, only to find a high reading the next time I measured.

Ketoacidosis

Hyperglycaemia, as discussed in Chapter 2, is high blood glucose. If your glucose gets very high there is a danger of diabetic ketoacidosis. After nine years of fairly good control (an average HbA1C of between 7 and 8[1]), and (embarrassingly) having a written a self-help booklet on living with diabetes, I had an episode of keto-acidosis. Following my final exams at university, predictably I got quite drunk, and (not so predictably) was asleep by the afternoon. I had had lunch, but was too drunk to take insulin at the time. I woke up at midnight and vomited. By this point confusion was setting in and I was absolutely exhausted. As I was feeling sick, I thought it was better not to take any insulin, which was a bad idea. My blood glucose at this point was about 13mmol/L, but I reasoned that if I couldn't eat it was better not to inject. Technically I would have been all right if I had taken my Lantus®, but I didn't. I spent the rest of the night half-awake having bizarre and confused dreams, throwing up every two hours. By eight in the morning the nausea had subsided and my blood glucose level was still about 13mmol/L. I started to feel better if not well. I thought I had just drunk too much, too quickly and had made a fool of myself. However, at one in the afternoon the vomiting began again, and I realised that this wasn't just a normal hangover! I ended up admitting myself to hospital that afternoon. I declared myself as diabetic,

KETOACIDOSIS AHEAD

[1] This is a measure of your average blood sugar level.

and stated that I hadn't taken any insulin recently as I'd been throwing up. I was treated very quickly, and after an hour or so of being on insulin and saline drips felt quite a bit better! I was kept in hospital for 24 hours in total to monitor my levels. Before I was treated, though, I had thrown up nine times in 18 hours and felt awful. I would not recommend it, not even as research for a helpful booklet…!

Seriously, though, it was quite a shock. Not only was it a fairly horrendous experience, but it was surprising how easy it was to slip into such a state. It was the first time since diagnosis that I felt I had a serious disease, and the episode really brought home to me the importance of keeping on top of my diabetes. It's strange to think that even as a well-controlled diabetic, there lies beneath the surface the possibility of a total meltdown.

So what had gone wrong? Well, when the body is short of insulin the cells begin to starve since there is no sugar reaching them. At this point the body switches to a less efficient method to get energy. Not only does this produce less energy, but as a by-product ketones are left in the blood. These are poisonous chemicals (technically, oxidised secondary alcohols if you're interested), since they turn your blood acidic. It is this that makes you feel so bad.

Ketoacidosis is a serious and life-threatening condition. So if your blood glucose is over 15 mmol/L and you do not feel well **you must take action**. If you have consistently high blood sugar, test your urine by peeing on a Keto-Diastix™ which you should have been given on diagnosis. Another indicator is if your breath or urine smells strange - according to the medical establishment 'like pear-drops'. If the test strip indicates ketones are present and you feel unwell call the ambulance. They will treat you by putting you on a drip and giving you insulin. It is a highly serious condition and should be treated with the utmost urgency. If you have a meter that measures blood ketones then please see page 71 which provides guidelines on measuring blood ketones.

Symptoms of Ketoacidosis[1]
- a loss of appetite
- nausea or vomiting (feeling or being sick)
- a high temperature
- stomach pain and
- a fruity smell from your urine and/or your breath, which may smell like pear drops or nail varnish remover

Remember you may need to get medical advice urgently if your blood glucose and ketones are both high.

Less severe hyperglycaemia (blood glucose below 15 mmol/L and only mild symptoms) is not so serious. It is worth noting that caffeinated drinks do not seem to help hyperglycaemia, and in my experience actually seem to raise blood sugar levels when you're in this condition. To actively take away the horrible feeling of hyperglycaemia, I've found that a large amount of anti-oxidants (like Vitamin E) helps.

Anti–oxidants

I am not entirely certain how they work and so can only suggest you experiment with them when you have high blood glucose. The basic principle of it is that when you are hyperglycaemic, oxidants are produced in the blood. Oxidants are required in small amounts by the body to kill germs, but many more are produced than is necessary when you are hyperglycaemic and it is these oxidants that make you feel tired and groggy. Therefore, the body requires a reducing agent (sorry for the chemistry!) but it has to be mild since the body is a very delicate system.

Another name for a mild reducing agent is an anti-oxidant. A large dose should take away the majority, if not all, of the 'groggy' feeling in a fast

[1]http://www.nhsdirect.wales.nhs.uk/small/en/home/healthencyclopaedia/d/diabetestype1/symptoms

time (roughly 2 minutes or less) - quicker than a substantial injection of insulin. **But anti-oxidants do not lower the blood glucose level – you will still need to take extra insulin or lower it some other way.**

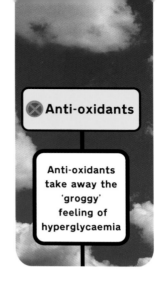

Anti-oxidants are found naturally in fruit, vegetables, and some teas. As a basic guide, a large bowl of salad or two cups of tea have roughly half the effect, in terms of taking away the 'groggy' feeling, as as a large dose of anti-oxidant pills. If you take the tea option, make sure that it is black, since the milk negates the effects of the anti–oxidants. As an important footnote, anti–oxidants and paracetamol can artificially raise the blood glucose reading on your machine: my personal estimate is by approximately 5 mmol/L. Therefore, if you have taken any anti–oxidants within the half hour before measuring, it is probably necessary to adjust the reading accordingly. You can find out how anti-oxidants affect your levels by measuring before and after taking them.

Injections and testing

Depending on which system you are on, you will be injecting either twice or four times a day. This is (literally sometimes!) a pain. If your injections are hurting you, think about the possible reasons why (apart from the fact that you are stabbing yourself with a piece of metal). These could include the brand of needle, since different manufacturers use different coatings on the needles which can irritate the skin. The needle could be too big or too small. You could also change the site of injection if you find it painful.

Generally speaking though, after a while, injections are not too much of a problem. The trick is finding what needle suits you and where to inject. In my case, on the four-a-day system, I use BD Microfine 8mm (31G) needles (a standard size as far as I'm aware). For breakfast I inject into the bottom of my right thigh, for lunch into the left side of my stomach, for dinner on the right side of the stomach and for the evening dose into the bottom of my left thigh.

It is important, especially on the four-a-day regime, to vary the injection site; on two-a-day it is less important but still recommended. This is because if you inject into the same area too frequently the body reacts and builds up a fatty deposit (a 'lump' – technical term!) at the injection site. This deposit, apart from looking and feeling a bit horrible, slows down the rate of insulin absorption and so lessens your immediate control. If you already have one of these 'lumps' then stop using that site and it will disappear within a couple of weeks.

Like most things with diabetes, taking injections is just something you have to get used to. If one injection does hurt (say you've hit a nerve, a blood vessel or you're using a 'dud' needle, and trust me, you will know!) just remove the pen (or syringe), change the site and possibly the needle and start again; there is no point in putting yourself through pain for no reason other than laziness.

The best sites to go for are the ones with the most amount of subcutaneous ('beneath the skin') fat. These include the stomach, the thighs, the bottom, and the back or side of your arms, and are where the insulin is absorbed at the most controlled rate. The technique of injection depends on what length of needle you are using to inject with. With long or medium length needles (8mm long or longer) you should 'pinch up' the skin around where you are injecting to make sure the needle goes into the subcutaneous fat and not the

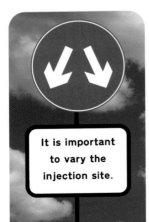

It is important
to vary the
injection site.

skin or muscle. With short needles you do not need to do this. All it comes down to is a matter of preference, although personally I go for pinching up since I find it makes injecting easier, but it makes no difference diabetically speaking.

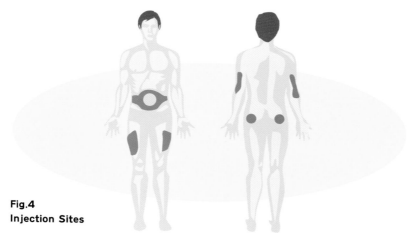

Fig.4
Injection Sites

If you have very little fat on your body your healthcare team should be able to give advice on any special technique you require to deliver the insulin correctly.

Blood glucose testing is similar to insulin injections since they can both be painful and tedious. If you do not measure regularly, you will not feel bad as a direct consequence, and you will not feel poorly immediately as you would if you did not inject your insulin when you needed to. However, you are more likely to feel bad as an indirect consequence: you will be less likely to know how much insulin you should take, and not knowing your blood glucose level makes it hard to take the appropriate measures to keep it under control.

Eventually you may be able to notice certain feelings and make an educated guess at your blood glucose level. However, this 'expertise' can take a long time to acquire, and still the only way you can learn accurately is to measure your blood glucose level when you get certain feelings and then either remember it or note it down. Writing down your results will also help you pick up strange factors that affect your glucose levels. For example, I've worked out that showers seem to raise my blood sugar level slightly since I've very rarely had a reading lower than 10mmol/L after having one. Once you note these kinds of factors down you can begin to associate certain feelings and events with different glucose levels.

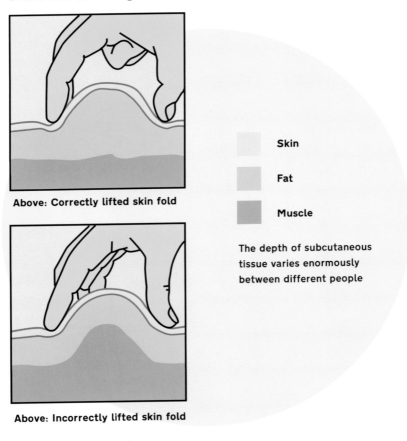

Above: Correctly lifted skin fold

Skin

Fat

Muscle

The depth of subcutaneous tissue varies enormously between different people

Above: Incorrectly lifted skin fold

Fig.5 Injection Methods

Since I have advised measuring as much as possible, I must recommend using a measuring device that works on blood not solely from the fingers. The machines that just take measurements from the

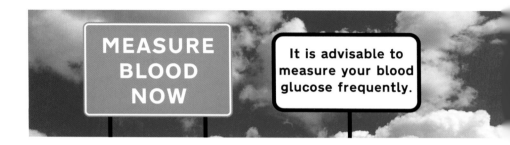

fingers are fine in the way that they are very accurate (usually with a degree of error less than 0.4 mmol/L either way) but they are troublesome since there is a limited amount of space on your fingers for you to lance and draw blood. I found that by lancing the side of the fingertips it was much less painful than on the pad, which is very sensitive.

This also saves some of the sensitivity in your fingers. Remember too, if you are using a device that measures the blood from the fingers, to draw blood to your hands before you lance a finger by shaking your hands and squeezing the blood to the tip of the selected finger.

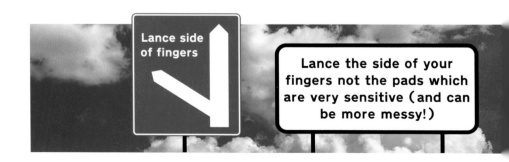

If you are measuring a lot though – four or more times a day – it is worth speaking to your healthcare team about getting a machine that can take measurements from the blood in your arms (sometimes called an 'alternate site meter'). They are slightly less accurate (my present meter is accurate to 0.4 mmol/L) but are far less painful and can save your fingers. This is especially important considering that it is often the extremities (fingers and toes specifically) that suffer first from poor diabetic control. You should be able to get one of these meters on the National Health Service.

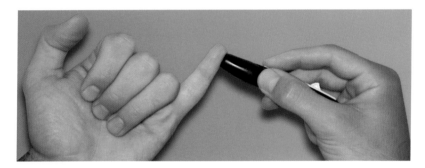

Fig.6 Lancing technique using the finger.

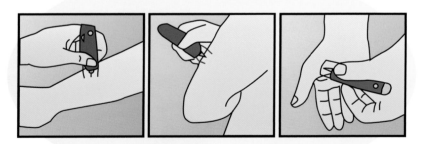

Fig.7 Lancing technique using the arms or the base of the thumb

Balancing your insulin with your food intake

As you know, because you have Type 1 diabetes you need to take insulin every day and several times a day to compensate for the fact that your body does not make its own. The key to good diabetic control is matching your insulin dosage with your food intake, exercise level and other lifestyle factors so that your blood glucose always (well… nearly always) stays within certain limits. Your diabetes team will tell you the limits that are right for you, but in general blood glucose levels should be 4 mmol/L to 7 mmol/L before meals and 2 hours after a meal go no higher than 11 mmol/L.

▼
7.0
4.0
▲

In general blood glucose levels should be 4.0 mmol/L to 7.0 mmol/L before meals and go no higher than 11.0 mmol/L two hours after a meal. Check with your diabetes team for your own personal 'targets'.

So how do you achieve the magic 'perfect control' ? The starting point is the insulin regimen prescribed by your diabetes specialist. The specialist you have seen has considerable experience in treating people with diabetes and will have prescribed the regimen he/she thinks is best for you, but as I said before, you have to self-medicate, and ultimately it is you who is in control of your blood glucose. I shall describe how I have managed my control and hope that what I have learned will give you a few tips to help you to adjust your food/lifestyle/insulin to obtain the best possible control for you.

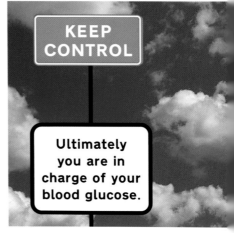

KEEP CONTROL

Ultimately you are in charge of your blood glucose.

Insulin regimens

I started on the insulin lispro (Humalog® M25™ Lilly) system, which meant two injections a day – one before breakfast and one before dinner. However, this system requires you to have a mid-morning snack, lunch, and a snack before bedtime. Not only did I find this inflexible, requiring me to plan almost everything I was going to eat during the day when I woke up (literally), but also very fattening, since I had to eat frequently and when I didn't necessarily want to. Children are advised to stick to the two-a-day regimen because their lives are more regimented and controlled than those of older people.

I would, therefore, highly recommend to any adolescent or older person with diabetes, if they are not already on it, to switch to the four injections a day system. The insulin I use now is the long-acting 24 hour, slow-release insulin glargine (Lantus®, Aventis) which I take at night, and the short–acting insulin lispro (Humalog® M100™ Lilly), which I take before breakfast, lunch and dinner. The brilliant thing about this regimen is the comparative flexibility. The Humalog® is so quick that you can even take it after a meal to no real detriment (this might not be medically advised but sometimes there is no opportunity to inject beforehand). Theoretically, you can even skip meals altogether and not take any insulin, but I have never done this and would not advise it. The great advantage of this system, due to its flexibility, is that you can eat when and what you want, not just when your regimen demands it. This also means that you can tailor your insulin dose more accurately, since you take smaller more frequent doses each time, as opposed to two bulk loads on the other system, and you can take into account other factors such as exercise (Chapter 4), alcohol (Chapter 5) or heat (Chapter 6), on the spur of the moment. To be able to use this system well, though, you have to know what you are doing, in a diabetic sense, which is where this guide should help.

As a basic guide to how much insulin you should take (on average) per day, an adult should take about 1 unit of insulin per kg of body weight. An adolescent should take about 1 – 1.5 units of insulin per kg of body weight (this difference is due to the effect of hormone levels which differ in adolescents and adults).

The Routine

Having just sung the praises of a flexible insulin regimen it may seem strange for me to suddenly argue for a fixed routine. However, it is the best way to keep control, and the four-a-day system simply means it is easier to break your routine and keep control: but just because you can be erratic doesn't mean you should be.

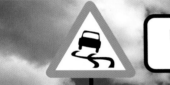

If you stray from the routine you are less likely to be in control.

Starting a new routine is always difficult because the only way to perfect it is through trial and error, and the trouble is that the routine shifts around, since when it is hot you require less insulin, and when it is cold you require more; if you are inactive or ill you require more whereas if you exercise regularly you will need less.

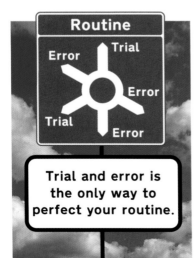

Trial and error is the only way to perfect your routine.

But as an example, by this method I worked out that in August (average temperature 25°C a day) I required 24 units of Lantus® a day and 1 unit of Humalog® M100™ for every 5g of carbohydrate I ate. However, remember this is what was right for me at the time – I was quite inactive then – and this may well not be the same for everyone. The important thing is to establish a basic routine to go back to that you can adjust slightly if necessary.

It is a good idea to write down your routine. This is probably most important for a person newly diagnosed with diabetes since it is very easy to forget certain aspects of the routine until they become second nature (which they will).

Sorting out your own routine is a subjective matter, and to help, I have included a carbohydrate index of foods (see Chapter 10).

When starting a routine I would highly advise checking the back of food packets for carbohydrate levels and even in some cases, such as cereals, weighing out the amount of food and calculating the amount of carbohydrate present. This should help you get your insulin bearings and will soon get you started on a well-controlled routine. You will gradually learn the carbohydrate content of various foods; for example, I know that a thick-sliced piece of wholemeal bread is roughly 15g of carbohydrate.

Remember that the food you eat makes all the difference to your health. Also, you shouldn't take extra insulin for the fat and protein in food. In fact, if you do take them into consideration, you should probably take less insulin. This is because fats and proteins are absorbed very, very slowly, meaning that their energy doesn't really raise the blood glucose level, and also that the stomach is kept fuller for longer in comparison with carbohydrates.

If you have worked out your routine and you stick to it more or less you will not go far wrong. It is only when we are weak-willed and don't stop to think that things can start to go out of control: ("One more biscuit/doughnut/ice-cream/beer/glass of wine/packet of crisps won't hurt!") The trouble is, if you haven't accounted for it then it will 'hurt', or complicate matters at any rate. I know this approach sounds tedious, over-meticulous, and petty, but – it works! Being petty is also a small sacrifice to make to ensure you live your full term of life and (with any luck) have a high quality of living.

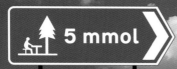

Being petty may mean you live longer and live better!

Using an insulin pump

I personally did not want to have an insulin pump installed. The needle is inserted and left in place for about three days. After that the injection site is changed, as with single injections. They work in a similar way to my current four-a-day injection system, but obviously with a lower frequency of injections! The important difference is that the pump only contains short-acting insulin. You set a base rate, which pumps a constant low level of insulin into the body, and then take extra 'hits' of insulin as and when you need to eat (as with my current Humalog®).

The two methods are just as flexible in terms of controlling glucose levels, and it really comes down to a balance between cost and treatment. Modern pumps are very effective in their treatment of diabetes: they are all

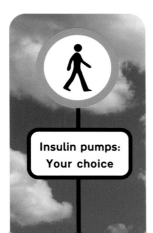

Insulin pumps: Your choice

robust and some are even waterproof. However, to stay on the safe side you may want to remove it if you are playing a contact sport or swimming. When insulin pumps are harnessed with Continuous Glucose Monitoring (CGM), where a small sensor is inserted under your skin that constantly checks your glucose levels, they are probably the best treatment available. The only real problem with these systems is cost. They are not generally available on the NHS; the cheapest pumps are around £850.

Please don't let my decision not to pump affect you, I just 'like' the injections! When it comes down to it, the decision to pump is highly individual, and if it works for you then that's great. All I would say is discuss your options with your diabetes team. Don't worry, if you use a pump my advice still applies!

Glycaemic Index (GI) and Insulin Index (II)

The Glycaemic Index (GI) shows how rapidly certain foods are absorbed into the body. Foods with a high GI raise blood glucose quickly; those with a low GI cause a slow and gradual rise in glucose.

Some forms of high GI carbohydrate, such as those in potatoes and in white bread, are absorbed nearly as rapidly as the carbohydrate in refined sugar. Diabetes is all about keeping control and so obviously the GI is significant. The most important use of GI comes in understanding your fluctuations. For example, if you know that you've just eaten some food with a high GI, then it is to be expected that the blood glucose will be relatively high and that you may feel some related symptoms, before the insulin you have injected brings it down. However, the insulin will only bring the blood glucose level down if you have taken enough. If you know your Insulin Index (the amount of carbohydrate that is put into cells by one unit of insulin), you can calculate how much insulin it takes to put that quantity of carbohydrate into the cells. Therefore, in normal day-to-day life, the Glycaemic Index is best used in conjunction with the Insulin Index.

The Glycaemic Index has a position subservient to the Insulin Index. At the end of the day, if you know that you've taken enough insulin but still have high blood glucose because of recently eating a high GI food, then you know that you don't have to take any more insulin. Taking more insulin could cause complications such as going hypo, then over-compensating with food, taking too much insulin, going hypo – the cycle would continue.

Unfortunately, this hard and fast advice is not always applicable. In some cases, particularly with fruit and some vegetables, the low GI of these foods seems to affect the Insulin Index. It seems to be due mainly to the fibre content slowing up absorption, as far as I can tell.

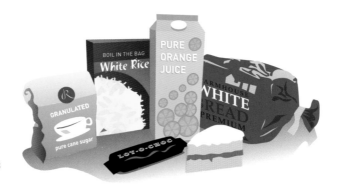

Fig.8

Above - High GI foods: Sugar, Rice, White bread, Chocolate bar, Cake, Fruit juice
Below - Low GI foods: Whole grain bread, Baked beans, Meat, Fish, Chicken

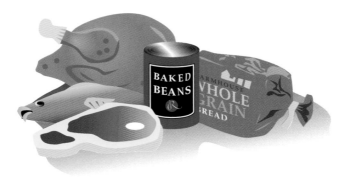

For example, a can of baked beans (50g of carbohydrate) should, according to my calculations, take 10 units of insulin to keep the blood glucose steady. However, it actually takes about half as much insulin as the carbohydrate is absorbed so slowly. I have found a similar effect with apricots, but please don't take my word for it – experiment!

The other main important point about the Glycaemic Index is knowing what you should eat or drink when hypo. This is relatively straightforward: ingest a high GI substance to raise the blood glucose as quickly as possible. However, you should try to keep a count of how much carbohydrate you are taking. This is more difficult than it sounds, and in time you will be able to estimate how much carbohydrate you need to treat an 'average' hypo (if there is such a thing). As ever, the importance here lies in testing, before and after the hypo.

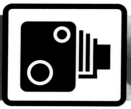

It is important to test before and after food, exercise etc to find out the effect on your blood glucose.

Working out your Insulin Index

You should try to work out how much a chosen amount of carbohydrate raises your blood glucose level, and over what period of time. This can be especially helpful in the delicate juggling act that is diabetic life. For example, I know that a slice of wholegrain bread (approx. 15g of carbohydrate) will raise my blood glucose level by about 8 mmol/L approximately an hour after eating it (without taking insulin or having it on top of a meal that I know I have taken the right amount for). Knowing when you've taken the exactly right the amount is difficult to work out though. Effectively, it can only be discovered through trial and error, a lot of measuring, and thinking about what other factors could have affected your blood sugar level. It might also be worth writing down the results in a diary. It's a bit tedious but after you've learnt how everything affects you (insulin, activity, climate etc.) you wouldn't have to use it anymore.

By this method I worked out the 'magic' ratio of 5g of carbohydrate:1 unit of Humalog® (this will probably not be perfect for you but it may be a good base for starting your experiment). I also worked out that if my blood glucose was too high, every extra unit of insulin I took would lower the level by roughly 2.7 mmol/L.

Here is my Insulin Index calculation:
15 g carbohydrate = 8 mmol/L rise in blood glucose

15 g carbohydrate = 3 units of insulin

Therefore 3 units of insulin will lower blood glucose by 8 mmol/L

And 1 unit will lower blood glucose by 8/3 = 2.6666 mmol/L

I hope you can see that working out the Insulin Index is essential to accurate control and is, in my opinion, the most important piece of information in this guide. Once you have worked this out for yourself, for normal living, you can adapt it, with an educated guess, to any different lifestyle you encounter and you should be able to achieve near-perfect control.

To achieve this high level of control it is best if you carry your diabetic equipment (insulin pen, glucose meter, needles, sensors and spare lancets) around with you all the time, along with some emergency food (see p.60). This way you can work out where your blood glucose is and treat it intelligently. It's a bit of a hassle to carry around all this stuff, but it's worth it in terms of the level of control you can achieve.

If your control isn't 'near-perfect' (and let's face it, whose is?) here is some advice for when things go a bit wrong. If you've got high blood sugar before a mealtime there are two main tricks to help to bring it back down to a normal level.

If you're taking a small amount of extra insulin to knock the level down, you have to wait about 10 - 20 minutes to allow it to work. Otherwise, the extra dose seems to get 'lost' and has no real effect. If you're taking a large amount of extra insulin (5 units or more), you should be all right to eat immediately. However, if you've got a blood glucose level that requires that much to bring it down you probably won't be that hungry!

The second trick is to eat a very slow release (low GI) meal, as that way you can take the insulin and eat straightaway. You'll still need to take excess insulin to deal with the extra glucose in your blood, but at least you can eat immediately. I've found that a particularly good meal in these kinds of situations is baked beans and tuna or scrambled eggs. Not the most sociable of meals perhaps, but very useful for control. You can reproduce its benefits by having a meal of protein (meat, fish or eggs) and a lot of vegetables and a small amount of carbohydrate (one slice of bread at most).

4. EXERCISE

Exercise is a key aspect of remaining fit and healthy. Being a person with diabetes, it is especially important since all those minor lapses in control make you far more susceptible to disease and illness. Exercise is also important in making you feel better since not only are endorphins (the body's natural opiates) released just after exercise, but it can also help improve your immune system, your self-image, self-confidence, and therefore your social skills.

The downside to it though is that it complicates your diabetic control. Exercise has the same effect as insulin in that it lowers the blood glucose level by inducing glucose to be transported into the cells. Therefore the amount and intensity of exercise has to be taken into consideration before you begin, and it is highly advisable to measure your blood glucose as well.

On my current insulin dosage routine I have worked out that running, on a treadmill in the gym, at 8 mph for 14 minutes, which burns 250 kCal (according to the machine), lowers my blood glucose level by about 5 mmol/L approximately half an hour after exercise. This involved measuring immediately before exercise, and several times afterwards. Remember that prolonged exercise can work on lowering blood glucose for many hours afterwards - the muscles store glucose as glycogen, and prolonged exercise uses this up. When you are at rest the body replaces these glucose stores, lowering your blood sugar level.

I know that a long jog (an hour or more) can lower my blood sugar level well into the next day if I run in the afternoon. If you go running like this almost every day, the effect builds up so that your glucose levels are constantly lowered. It is worth pointing out here that you should artificially raise your glucose levels before doing exercise – you don't want to be halfway through a long jog only to realise you're hypo with no way of helping yourself. It's a good idea to take a GlucoGel® with you when you go running, or maybe a fast-acting sugar source like a Boost® bar to the gym. People may give you funny looks when they see you bring chocolate or sweets into the gym, but they are preferable to the looks you'd get in a coma!

Also, depending upon the exercise you're doing, you'll probably get different readings after a workout. For example, an hour-long weights session doesn't seem to lower glucose as readily as an hour of cardiovascular activity like running. This is probably just because you'll use up more energy exercising your legs for an hour than even a large upper body muscle group like your chest.

For me, 50 kCal of energy used equates to the lowering of blood glucose by 1 mmol/L. Therefore 125 kCal used is roughly equivalent to 1 unit of Humalog® insulin. I can use this ratio to see how much exercise I need to take to lower my blood glucose by a certain amount. Do you see a pattern emerging yet?! It is this kind of thinking that enables greater control and indirectly will keep you alive and healthier for longer.

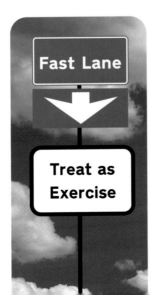

Sex

Let's face it, if you're exercising well, you're going to be looking good and are more likely to get some action. Sex is one of those incentives to keep you alive and healthier for longer. Like any other aspect of life, though, you have to be able to think about it diabetically. Sex has a similar effect upon blood glucose as any other form of exercise. However, it is obviously a bit more awkward to measure your glucose levels before and after, as it could be described as a 'bit of a mood-killer'! Also, it is less easy to estimate how each 'session' will affect your blood sugar, unless you're doing the same thing each time, to the same intensity etc. My only advice is to treat it like exercise (diabetically, at least!) and raise your blood sugar level slightly beforehand to a level of around 10mmol/L. That way you won't have to stop for a pee because of hyperglycaemia, or for some food because of hypoglycaemia. How will you know you're at this level? I'm sure you'll find a way: necessity is the mother of invention! It is also worth mentioning that, along with the usual symptoms, if you're a male with a hypo you might find it more difficult to 'perform'.

Losing weight

The following information is essential to losing weight and remaining healthy as a diabetic. By running regularly over a 2 month period and eating less I lost between 1 and 1.5 stones (7-10 kgs).

As a person with diabetes it is very easy to put on weight, even if you do exercise. Not only does your healthcare team encourage a high carbohydrate diet but insulin actually encourages your appetite as well (which is why, when you try to lower high blood glucose with insulin, it can be a test of self-control as well as self-knowledge!). If you exercise but do not take into account its glucose-lowering effect, then you will simply end up eating more, and probably more high-energy food to deal with the hypos that could occur, leading to weight-gain.

The way to lose weight when you are a diabetic is to lower your insulin dosage. This will lower your appetite, not only because there will be less insulin in your system but also because raised levels of blood glucose are an appetite suppressant as well. This does not mean you should stop taking your insulin as this could cause DKA, and accelerate the onset of devastating complications. To deal with these slightly raised levels you need to take regular exercise, eat fruit and vegetables and drink black tea (for their anti-oxidant effects). Also, you should eat a higher proportion of protein and drink plenty of water. The water will not only rehydrate you but also fill you up. The protein will be needed by the body for the repair and growth of the muscles you will be using exercising. However, the protein is also an appetite suppressant since it takes a very long time to be digested in the stomach. I have found from personal experience that a fairly large tuna salad (200g of tuna, 1/3 of a green pepper, 1/3 of a red pepper, 1/2 a lettuce, 1/5 of a cucumber and French salad dressing) will keep me feeling physically full for about 3 hours.

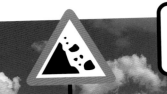

The way to lose weight when you are a diabetic is to lower your insulin dosage.

As a good general note, if you have eaten a lot of protein or a large meal the high GI foods will be absorbed less quickly. This is handy if you want a dessert and don't want to raise your blood glucose too quickly, but it can also be dangerous since you might go hypo and not be able to deal with it in time. As ever, just think before you eat! For example routines see Chapter 8.

You should consult your doctor before changing your diet and exercise routine. Also, joining a gym is a good idea as not only will other people be around to help if you suddenly go hypo when exercising but the instructor should also be able to structure a routine suitable for you. You should also build up your fitness slowly. This means listening to your body, a skill, that as a diabetic, you will almost definitely develop: not pushing your body too far whilst still pushing it enough! With diabetes it's all about keeping things level - hence the name of the Diabetes UK flagship magazine - Balance.

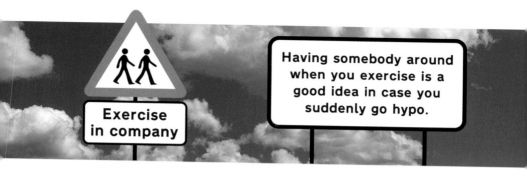

Exercise in company

Having somebody around when you exercise is a good idea in case you suddenly go hypo.

5. DRUGS

Having said that diabetes is all about balance and control, drugs are all about imbalance and lack of control. Of course, they come in many different shapes, forms and levels of disharmony within the body. This booklet is simply to advise: from a diabetic standpoint you should probably avoid them all, as any person should. However, normal people do not avoid all drugs by any means, and as you are diabetic you should just know how you are affecting your body so that you know what, and what not, to worry about, when taking a drug.

Cigarettes

I know you've heard it before, but you really shouldn't smoke these, or do anything with them, come to that! So how do they affect you as a diabetic? Well, the nicotine releases fats and sugars into your blood, much like adrenaline, and so raises your blood glucose level. Over time this causes the blood vessels to become stickier and blood more likely to clot. When you take into consideration that high blood glucose causes much the same as this, it means that you are far more likely to suffer the effects of high blood glucose in your extremities: lower blood flow leads to loss of feeling, possibly impotence, and a higher likelihood of heart disease. The nicotine is highly addictive, supposedly more so than cocaine, and so starting smoking is a very bad idea since the amount usually increases rapidly and is very hard to stop.

STOP THINK ACT

If you are diabetic you should know
how drugs affect your body
so that you know what, or what not,
to worry about.

The tar in inhaled tobacco smoke kills the cells in the throat causing the infamous smoker's cough. It also destroys the delicate cells in your lungs making breathing harder. It isn't a particularly pleasant smell either and could be called (by a significant minority) anti-social.

In addition, smoking lowers your immune system and so makes it more likely that you will be ill, something to be avoided at all costs if you are diabetic as it means a change in routine, which is troublesome in the short term and damaging in the long term.

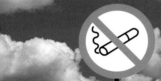

**Smoking is not a good idea
for people with diabetes**

Alcohol

It is very important when drinking alcohol to remember that it lowers the blood glucose level. Basically, alcohol temporarily stops the liver from converting glycogen (stored carbohydrate) into glucose. This means that no new glucose will be put into your blood system unless you eat, meaning that you can quite quickly go hypo. To combat this I would advise either taking less insulin before you drink, and/or eating during or after drinking. The first of these options may leave you with a high blood glucose feeling for up to an hour (which is not comfortable) but it is safer than the second method. This is because you may drink too much and not be physically able to eat anything to bolster your blood glucose level.

The amount your blood glucose changes is a direct consequence of the type of alcohol you are drinking. Almost all alcoholic drinks contain some form of carbohydrate. Beers are quite starchy, at around 4% carbohydrate. It doesn't sound like a lot, but 4% of a pint of beer (568ml)[1] is about 22 grams of carbohydrate – the equivalent of a thickly sliced piece of bread. After drinking a fairly large amount

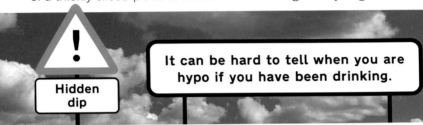

Hidden dip

It can be hard to tell when you are hypo if you have been drinking.

of beer (five pints or more) your blood glucose can rocket up to above 20 mmol/L. The case is similar with alcopops which are obviously sweet. In comparison, wine raises blood glucose very slightly and spirits not at all, before all of them lower it. I'm not advising you to cut out beer and alcopops from your diet, but just to realise and understand the consequences of drinking them. Generally speaking, in these 'beery' circumstances I take an extra dose of insulin before I go to bed to bring my blood glucose to a level of around 10 mmol/L, and then count on the alcohol to lower it another 5mmol/L or so for the morning. I could lower it further but it's better to place your blood sugar in slightly raised 'safer' limits in these scenarios just in case you go miscalculate and go hypo.

The alcohol industry is now producing sugar-free varieties of alcopops and mixers (such as diet Red Bull) which are, in normal drinking circumstances for a diabetic, obviously preferable. However, if you are

[1] http://www.calorieking.com/foods/calories-in-beer-regular-5-alc_f-Y2lkPTM5NT gwJmJpZD0xJmZpZD02MTMwNSZwYXI9.html

also dancing a lot in a club it is probably a good idea to use the sweet varieties, as the alcohol and exercise work together to lower your blood glucose level. It can also be quite hard to tell when you are hypo if you are drunk or have been drinking. In my opinion it is probably better to err on the side of caution and take less insulin, eat more or (unpopularly) drink less.

But how do you know where the line of caution is before you've crossed it? Well, that's the hard part. Trial and error is the only true way to work it out, and it's probably best to start experimenting with wine, or spirits if you really want to. Beer's starchiness complicates matters and makes it difficult to work out how much it affects your blood glucose level. I now know that a standard glass of 12% wine (175ml, roughly 2 units of alcohol) will lower my sugar level by about 4 mmol/L over the course of approximately 2 hours. Therefore, one glass of wine is as effective as 1.5 units of Humalog® at lowering the blood sugar level (but considerably slower). From this experience I now know that 1 unit of alcohol will lower my blood glucose by about 2 mmol/L. If I apply this information to beer you see that, even if it is 5%, it won't lower the glucose level overall.

1 pint of 5% alcohol beer= 22g of carbohydrate, and 3 units of alcohol.

In my current routine 22g of carbohydrate will raise my blood glucose by about 12 mmol/L. 3 units of alcohol will lower it by about 6 mmol/L. By the end of the evening you can see that the blood sugar level would probably be quite high after a few pints. However, it is worth noting that, like heavy exercise, heavy drinking can keep lowering your blood sugar level through to the next day. Try and keep this in mind as you deal with your hangover!

So from this you can work out how much more you need to eat or how much less insulin you have to take. In this respect it is much like any other aspect of diabetic control and I strongly advise you to keep a note of it if you are new to the disease (Welcome to the Club!) and even if you're not: thinking straight isn't most people's normal reaction to drinking, nor is memory improved by it – quite the reverse in fact!

Let's face it, drinking can get quite messy sometimes whether you're an old hand or a beginner.   This can be the scary part of drinking, especially if you are, or think you are, going hypo whilst feeling nauseous.   Thankfully, this has never happened to me, but if the situation does occur I advise taking a GlucoGel©, which is absorbed through the lining of the cheek, and calling the ambulance.

Unless you have a large stock of GlucoGel©, I would ring the paramedics immediately; they will probably put you on a drip with glucose in it. It is standard paramedic procedure - even 'normal' non-diabetic people can suffer from hypoglycaemia if they have drunk too much.

Cannabis
Taking cannabis is not advisable. As far as I know there is no confirmed evidence that it lowers the blood glucose level, but I think the two are probably linked due to the symptom known as 'the munchies', where users get very hungry after taking the drug.

Ecstasy, cocaine, heroin, LSD, magic mushrooms, speed, steroids
I just wouldn't. Not a good idea, just as cannabis isn't, due to a lack of knowledge of the effects of these drugs. Also, it puts you in the dangerous position of being high and going hypo and not caring or not being able to deal with it.

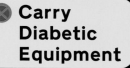

**Carry
Diabetic
Equipment**

Carry at least a GlucoGel and your insulin if you think you may want to stay over after a night out.

All these drugs are bad enough for non-diabetic people, and I'm not saying that you can't drink, you can't smoke, you can't take ecstasy, but as a diabetic it isn't such a good idea. If you do, though, you just have to work through the complications beforehand, know what you are doing and how it will affect you.

One of the reasons most people take drugs is to let off some steam, to lose control. As a diabetic you should never be totally out of control since this is when problems begin. In effect, lose control in a controlled manner – another of those brilliant diabetic acts that can make living very tiring! I would also advise that, as ever, you take your diabetic equipment around with you but at the very least a GlucoGel© and your insulin on a night out. You never know when you may want to crash at a friend's house, only to discover you can't, or at least shouldn't.

If you want more drug advice I suggest you visit: **www.talktofrank.com** or call them on **0800 77 66 00.** This is a government-sponsored site and it should be able to answer any of your queries satisfactorily.

6. TRAVELLING

Going travelling as a diabetic is, like most aspects of diabetic life, just a bit more complicated than for 'normal' people. I would advise making a checklist of your diabetic equipment (insulin, needles, syringes [for emergencies], pens, sensors, glucose meter and lancets) before you go away, and make sure you are well stocked. The best way to do this is to calculate how many needles and sensors you will need for your trip and then take half as many again, if not double. It might be a good idea to separate your diabetic supplies into two groups, in case one group is lost or stolen. This way you can almost rule out entirely the possibility of running out. You should also bring a spare insulin pen and excess insulin, just to be safe.

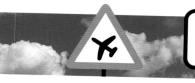

Take a spare insulin pen and excess insulin when travelling.

I strongly recommend storing the insulin in a refrigerated wallet whilst in transit and, as normal, in a fridge whilst on holiday, especially if it is hot. You should take your insulin around with you to ensure flexibility even if the weather is hot; nobody wants to spend their holiday feeling foul due to high blood glucose.

If travelling by aeroplane take your diabetic equipment with you as hand luggage. Firstly, you will probably need to inject during the flight for the in-flight 'meal'. Secondly, you do not want to arrive at your destination to discover your luggage with all your diabetic stuff (i.e. your life source) has been lost by an incompetent member of airport staff (yes, they do exist!) You do not need to worry about bringing needles on-board as hand-luggage, as I have done it (nervously) many times without a problem: they do not think you are a terrorist!

However, before leaving the country, it is probably advisable to obtain a doctor's note saying that you are diabetic. Also, you should probably inject in the loo in-flight as, although security might not think you are a terrorist, people can be quite squeamish about injections and there's no need to upset them.

A doctor's note confirming that you are a competent, well-controlled diabetic can be handy when travelling.

If you are travelling by ship, or 'boat' to us land-lubbers, remember to take into account that sea-sickness and rough weather may upset your stomach and lose you your lunch. My advice is to either not eat

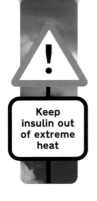

Keep insulin out of extreme heat

on ship or just before boarding, or to inject a little less insulin than required so that if the worst comes to the worst your blood glucose won't plummet horribly. It's never happened to me but I can imagine that sea-sickness and hypoglycaemia do not make for a fun time. If this does happen, treat it with a GlucoGel©.

If you are walking, hiking, swimming, cycling or climbing on holiday do not forget to take into account how much these activities may affect your blood glucose level.

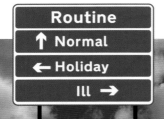

Routine

↑ Normal

← Holiday

Ill →

It may take some days to acclimatise to a change of routine on holiday.

Going on holiday is like any change of routine and as such it could take up to two weeks (or possibly more) to acclimatise to it. It is particularly for this reason that you should take extra insulin with you, in case you require more on a daily basis than you estimated, but also for unforeseen emergencies such as your transport being delayed by days. For these reasons you should take your own supply of sweets with you on holiday to deal with any hypos that occur in transit or during your stay. All of this depends upon the climate and how active you are on holiday, but it is best to make sure you are covered. You should also get medical travel insurance to safeguard yourself against the unexpected.

If you are planning on scuba diving, submarining, paragliding, bungee-jumping or even water-skiing you should almost definitely tell the person in charge that you are diabetic. This may stop you from doing that activity as their insurance may not cover you. By all means go against my advice if you want to but I do not believe it is worth the risk. Possibly a doctor's note, saying that you are a competent, well-managed diabetic would help, so I suggest you bring one with you.

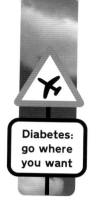

Diabetes: go where you want

Just like any other aspect of diabetic living, simply think ahead about how certain factors might affect you. For example, if it is hot you may require less insulin than usual. This will either be because you are less hungry in the heat or because increased blood-flow to the injection site may mean that the insulin is absorbed more quickly. Also, if you are on a beach holiday, you will probably be drinking more alcohol and swimming more than usual, both of which would reduce your insulin requirement. Other extreme environments can affect your blood glucose level as well; high altitude causes the body to use up more energy to respire.

You shouldn't worry too much about looking after your insulin in the heat (especially if you have a large reserve in a nearby fridge as I have advised). According to the major manufacturers of insulin (Eli Lilly, Novonordisk, Sanofi Aventis) in temperatures above 30°C you should try to keep it out of direct sunlight. Try and keep it in the shade or in your pocket, and don't leave it in the hot sun for hours as it might denature and stop working. However, don't let it stop you going to hot places. To err on the side of caution though, you can carry your pen(s) around in a Frio® Wallet when the weather is really hot, and you will be away from a fridge for a significant period of time (a week trekking in the desert or jungle, for example). If you don't have such a wallet it may be worth simply placing the insulin next to a bottle of water to keep it cool.

It is also worth remembering when travelling to far-off places to take into account the time difference. I wouldn't advise trying to work out when to take your long-acting insulin dose in your new time zone as this could complicate matters: you may need to take a Lantus® injection in the middle of the afternoon. On the day you leave home take the dose in the evening as usual, and take the next long-acting dose the next evening. This will cause complications as well, but ones that are perhaps easier to manage. For example, if the time between the doses is shorter than usual, you'll know to take less short-acting insulin during that period or be prepared to eat more!

Driving

First of all, the DVLA advises measuring every time before you drive, and not setting off before your blood glucose is over 5mmol/L. However, despite your best intentions glucose levels can fluctuate quite a bit so it's a good idea to take further precautions. Whenever you are driving always make sure that you have an emergency supply of sweets in the car. If you do go hypo, simply pull over at the nearest safe place and sort it out. This is especially important for young, inexperienced drivers (mainly learners) who may find the levels of concentration required tiring as the brain actually uses up quite a lot of energy, and so lowers your blood glucose.

If you are applying for a licence you must tick the 'diabetic' box; don't worry, they will still give it to you! If you have been diagnosed after having passed your test then I think, though you should check with the DVLA or your healthcare team at least, that you have to notify the DVLA and get a new licence. This is because as a diabetic driver there are a few restrictions. As far as I know, you are not allowed to drive an HGV (anything over 3 tonnes). Also your licence is only valid for 3 years and has to be renewed after that time. It's not all doom and gloom though as the renewal service is free and requires no new test. The DVLA simply needs to

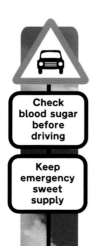

Check blood sugar before driving

Keep emergency sweet supply

make sure you're still fit to drive safely. Factors that could affect their decision are things like poor eyesight (due to retinopathy) and not being able to feel hypos any more. This second condition is obviously quite serious, even when you're not driving! Tell your doctor if you find this happening to you.

Drink driving

It's even worse for a diabetic due to the possible complication of a booze-induced hypo at the wheel. Imagine the situation: hands shaking, heart beat raised, confusion setting in and you're speeding to get home quickly to treat the hypo because you've forgotten your emergency supply in the car. It's just really stupid. Don't do it.

7. HOSPITAL, SCHOOL AND WORK

These three are probably the biggest influences on a diabetic's life, so it is important to know how to manage them.

Hospital

Depending on your age and health you will be required to go and see a diabetic specialist between one and four times a year. Some GP surgeries have their own but it is most likely that you will attend one at hospital. Whilst at the clinic a member of the team (most likely the diabetes nurse) will take your glycosylated haemoglobin level (HbA1C) This is a measure of how well your blood glucose has been controlled over the past 6-8 weeks. They will also measure your height, weight,

The diabetes team is there to help you.

and blood pressure. If there are any problems they will advise you how to deal with them and can set up appointments with a dietician or psychologist, or with a chiropodist if you have problems with your feet. In the adult clinic, which is less frequent than the children's, usually once a year, you will be required to have a blood test taken up to two weeks before the clinic, which will be used for testing things like thyroid and liver function. The adult version is a lot more thorough, in that they will test your eyes, inspect your feet, and take a urine sample during the same clinic. It is important to remember when at your clinic that the doctors and nurses only really want to help you, no matter how authoritarian they may appear. However, if you think they are wrong, or that their advice is not helpful, do not be afraid to tell them. You should be your own doctor on a day-to-day basis and, diabetically speaking, you should answer only to yourself. This position can only ever be achieved if you consistently have perfect results – which nobody does – but that does not mean it is not worth striving for. Also if you do attempt to argue with your team, make sure you are clear on all the facts and mechanisms of your diabetic control, otherwise you will be wrong, embarrassed and patronised for your poor understanding and control!

Seriously, the team is useful since they simply have more knowledge than you. You can, and should, ask them anything you want to know about diabetes and the various possible complications. If you do have any problems out of clinic time, say a chronic illness is diagnosed or you are worried about taking a trip somewhere because of your diabetes, you should call the diabetes nurses and they will talk to you or arrange tests for any problem you think you might have.

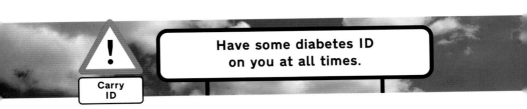

!
Carry ID

**Have some diabetes ID
on you at all times.**

As a related health issue, diabetics are more prone to illness in general – you should find that when you have high blood glucose you will feel worse and succumb to a disease quicker than when your diabetes is under control. You are also more likely to get thyroid complications since this is also an autoimmune disease like diabetes.

If you are ever brought conscious into a hospital you should make it known as soon as possible that you are diabetic. If you are brought in unconscious and without any ID you might slip into a coma, not a pleasant thought, so have some ID on you at all times and not just in your wallet: imagine if you were mugged and beaten up, for example.

If you are lucky, you will spend as little time as possible in hospital because you will probably be in one of the next two institutions – school or work.

School

If you were diagnosed while attending school you should let the teachers know as soon as possible. The school nurse should also be informed and given an emergency supply of GlucoGel© and sweets. If you ever go hypo whilst in a lesson and you think it really necessary, you should tell the teacher and they should let you go and deal with it. If they don't, persuade them with arguments such as "I can't be held responsible for any future actions", and "Do you think I'd be less disruptive in a coma on the floor?!" If they say "yes" to the second question, direct them towards the first argument!

Unfortunately, saying, "Can I go for a run, sir?" doesn't work for high blood glucose, so just get it right to begin with.

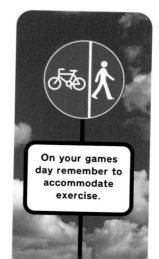

On your games day remember to accommodate exercise.

Lunch and break times can be a hassle, diabetically. Firstly, you should get permission to go into lunch whenever you need to and skip whatever queue exists if your blood glucose is low. If anyone tries to countermand this, refer them to the arguments above, but it might work to say: "This is my pay-off for having a disease for the rest of my life". Remember not to give in to temptation at the tuck-shop, servery or vending machines, and if you haven't taken enough insulin for an extra chocolate bar, don't have it, or simply take some more insulin – is it worth another jab?

On your games day remember to accommodate the exercise and take less insulin, or eat more, or do both, as long as you can work the high blood glucose off. For exams I recommend boosting your blood glucose 10 minutes or so beforehand as you really don't want to go hypo. If you are worried that high blood glucose will lessen your concentration you might want to just have some sweets with you and take them as and when you need to. In my opinion this is the riskier option; you don't want to be juggling diabetes with the finer points of Shakespeare under high pressure. Also if you can't concentrate in an exam, high blood glucose or not, there's not much chance for you; just push through it and you'll be surprised how much energy your brain uses up when taxed.

The only real bonus for diabetics comes in the form of GCSE Biology which contains diabetes as part of its syllabus. It's a given, so you should really have that one under your belt! Unfortunately, it's not that complicated at GCSE so it's not that much of an advantage, but a little less learning never hurt anyone (don't quote me on this!).

Work

Most of the things about school apply here too. Let all your colleagues know you're a diabetic, along with the company doctor or nurse if there is one. Remember that long-term stress has the same cardiovascular effects as smoking and high blood glucose, so try to avoid it. However, if you find that stress is unavoidable, you might find that taking a higher long-acting dose helps reduce your levels overall, rather than chasing 'hypers' with extra short-acting doses.

So there it is – simply a case of working out your routine and trying to stick to it. If you don't or can't – play it by ear and make an educated guess, or at worst learn from your mistakes. To avoid as many errors as possible there follows a section on working out the right insulin dose, and example routines for normal living, exercising and sickness. Please remember that these are only guidelines though, that you should use to help figure out how your body works, and take control, Your Way. If you have any problems get in touch with your healthcare team.

8. HOW TO WORK OUT HOW MUCH INSULIN TO TAKE

(1) **You have to work out how much insulin to take for a certain amount of carbohydrate. This can be a long and tricky process involving lots of measuring, so if you are very newly diagnosed it is probably best to estimate 1 unit of insulin to 5g of carbohydrate. This means that if you had 5g of carbohydrate you would need 1 unit of insulin to bring your blood sugar back to level. You should also work out by how much 5g of carbohydrate will raise your blood sugar level.** So, from a lot of measuring I know that under 'normal conditions' a slice of bread (15g of carbohydrate) will raise my blood sugar level by 8 mmol/L. Therefore, 5g of carbohydrate will raise my blood sugar level by 2.7 mmol/L. If there is a ratio of 1 unit of insulin:5g of carbohydrate, then 1 unit of insulin will lower my blood sugar level by 2.7 mmol/L.

② **You need to work out how much carbohydrate you are going to eat. You can estimate this, but if you want to be precise you can weigh the food and then divide this amount by its carbohydrate percentage (please see Chapter 10 for carbohydrate tables).**

So, a bagel is 40g of carbohydrate. In normal conditions I would need to take 8 units of insulin.

③ **Measure your blood sugar level. If it is too high you will want to lower it, if it is too low you will want to raise it. How are you going to do this? If you are planning on using insulin to do so, how much more or less will you have to inject?**

Let's say I've got a blood sugar of 15 mmol/L and I want to lower my blood sugar level to 5 mmol/L just with insulin. I know from step 1 that 1 unit of insulin will lower my blood sugar level by 2.7 mmol/L. Therefore, to lower my blood sugar by 10 mmol/L I will need to take either 3.5 or 4[1] extra units of insulin. If I'm having the bagel from step 2, I will inject 11.5 or 12 units.

If my blood sugar is 3.2 mmol/L I want to raise my blood sugar by about 5 mmol/L. Therefore, I will take 1.5 or 2 units less than I think I would normally need. If I'm having the bagel from step 2, I will inject 6.5 or 6 units.

④ **If I'm going to be doing some activity like drinking or taking exercise, I will adjust my dosage according to how much I think I will be doing.**

My blood sugar is 10 mmol/L, and I'm having a lasagne, which I estimate will be 60g of carbohydrate. Therefore, I should take 12 units of insulin. However, I'm drinking with my meal and think I'll have 2 glasses of wine (a total of 4 alcoholic units). From a lot of measuring I know that under 'normal conditions' that 1 unit of alcohol will lower my blood sugar level by 2 mmol/L. Two glasses of wine will lower my blood sugar by about 8 mmol/L, the equivalent of taking 3 units of

[1]For the purpose of these examples I am using an insulin pen with 0.5 unit divisions of dosage. With insulin pumps it is possible to be more accurate with the amount injected.

insulin, but after about 2 hours. Therefore, if I took 12 units of insulin the effect of the alcohol would make my blood sugar level go down to about 2 mmol/L. So instead I'll take 9 or 9.5 units of insulin so that my blood sugar should be about 8 mmol/L in a couple of hours' time.

Imagine the same scenario as above, except that instead of having wine I'll be drinking beer. I think I'll have 2 pints of 5% lager (a total of 6 alcoholic units). The beer is about 4% carbohydrate so 2 pints is a total of 44g grams of carbohydrate. I have to take some more insulin (9 units) to deal with all that extra carbohydrate from the beer. However, the alcohol will lower my blood sugar level by a further 12 mmol/L, or the same as taking 4.5 units of insulin, leaving my glucose dangerously low. This obviously isn't ideal. What I'll do then is take 4 to 4.5 units of insulin for the carbohydrate in the beer on top of the 12 units I'll take for the lasagne to make sure that my glucose level returns to a stable level.

Let's go back to that bagel. It's lunchtime, my blood sugar is 7 mmol/L and I've decided I'm going for a run later that afternoon. I plan on running for 15 minutes at 8 mph (roughly 250kCal), that should have the same effect on my blood sugar level as 2 units of insulin. There are a few ways of dealing with this situation. I can take 7 units of insulin for the bagel (when I should take 8) to raise my blood glucose to about 10 mmol/L for the run. The exercise will then lower my glucose level and I can take this into account in my next insulin dose for dinner. I can take 8 units and boost my blood sugar closer to the time I run with some extra carbohydrate. Both of these methods will result in the blood sugar being lowered below 7mmol/L after the run. Finally, I could plan for the amount of exercise I am going to do and its lowering effect in the lunchtime dose. So, in this final option I would only take 6 units of insulin for the bagel, but try to protect myself as much as possible by taking lots of anti-oxidants. However, I would recommend the first as the easiest to control and most comfortable out of these three options.

(5) **If the climate changes so that it becomes significantly hotter or colder, or if my glucose levels are consistently too high or too low I change the background insulin dose. This way you keep the important insulin:carbohydrate ratio effectively the same for working out how much short-acting insulin to take for each meal.**

So my blood sugar is constantly floating around or above 10 mmol/L before meals. I don't want to take extra short-acting insulin for each meal, which will change the 1 unit of insulin:5g carbohydrate ratio. I also don't want to have extra shots in between meals since they will complicate control, as the insulin in each injection is absorbed over a few hours. This means that extra injections will lead to greater fluctuations as the effect of an 'in between meal injection' can hangover to affect a standard injection. Therefore, I'll raise my Lantus® dose every day by 1 unit until my normal blood sugar level is closer to 5 mmol/L before meals. It doesn't sound like a massive difference but as I'm sure you'll appreciate, a small change in the way you treat diabetes can go a long way.

Example Routines:

Routine 1: Normal

Humalog Morning:	10 units bowl of fruit cereal with milk, (approx. 50g of carbohydrate), 1 cup of black coffee with 3 low calorie sweeteners
Humalog Lunch:	9 units ham, cheese, lettuce sandwich (approx. 30g of carbohydrate), pack of crisps (approx. 15g of carbohydrate)
Humalog Dinner:	12 units 4 slices of pizza (approx. 60g of carbohydrate), salad
Lantus Bed	24 units

Routine 2: Exercise / Weight Loss

Humalog Morning:	4 units
	2 slices of thick wholemeal bread with margarine and marmite (approx. 30g of carbohydrate), 1 cup of black coffee with 3 low calorie sweeteners
Exercise:	20 minutes running
Humalog Lunch:	3 units
	Tuna salad, 1 slice of toast with margarine and ham (approx. 15g of carbohydrate)
Humalog Dinner:	10 units
	roast chicken (not whole!), french beans, 2 baked potatoes (approx. 45g of carbohydrate), chocolate bar (approx. 15g of carbohydrate)
Lantus Bed	23 units

Routine 3: Cold / Illness

Humalog Morning:	12 units
	bowl of fruit cereal with milk, (approx. 50g of carbohydrate) 1 cup of black coffee with 3 low calorie sweeteners
Humalog Lunch:	13 units
	3 slices of thick wholemeal bread (approx. 45g of carbohydrate), 1 cuppa soup (approx. 15g of carbohydrate), 1 pint of water
Humalog Dinner:	10 units
	salmon steak, chips (approx. 45g of carbohydrate), salad
Lantus Bed	26 units

9. JOE'S SMALL-IN-ONE AND WHY I MADE IT

During my decade of diabetes I've come across a number of problems and tried to solve them as best I can. This booklet is simply my way of passing on the knowledge, know-how, and tricks that I've managed to pick up over the years. One of the things that I have found a constant nag, though, is carrying all the necessary diabetic equipment about. Often I would just have my short-acting insulin and a couple of needles on me (on top of the usual emergency glucose fix of a chocolate bar or two). This led to the inevitable problem of inflexibility and poor control – not a great advert for my way of dealing with diabetes.

The problem is that there is just so much stuff! Even if the glucose meter is small (and there are lots of small ones about these days), there is still the problem of carrying the finger-pricker, spare lancets, and pot of test-strips – and that's just for measuring. To be really flexible you need to have the short-acting insulin, but also the long-acting insulin pen, as well as more needles. On top of that, where can you put the used sharps and remain hygienic?

I suppose one answer to my problem would be a pump, and to be fair I haven't tried one. However, neither have the vast majority of diabetics, as pumps are expensive and not wholly supported by doctors. The answer is a bag for carrying all the stuff you need. Well, there are plenty of bags on the internet - believe me, I've looked. The trouble is they are either too large to be convenient to carry about or are too small to carry all the things I needed.

So I made Joe's Small-in-one, a carry case designed to be as convenient as possible. First of all, it's small – 16.5 x 10.5 x 3.8cm, or about the size of a glasses case. It carries all the diabetic equipment you should need for 24 hours' worth of treatment. This means you can just load it up in the morning and not worry about your supplies until the next day. It will hold

- 2 insulin pens
- 4 needles
- 1 glucose meter
- 1 finger pricker

- 1 pot of test-strips
- 4 spare lancets
- 1 packet of dextrose tablets
- Diabetic ID

Not only can it hold a lot, but more importantly it can carry a great variety of different meters and their accompanying test-strips and finger-prickers. Joe's Small-in-one can carry 18 of the 19 glucose meters available in Britain today[1], with the Prestige QX the only exception. On top of this, it's practical – made of durable, washable nylon, with a belt loop and an identification tag. So there you have it: a bag that's small, versatile, practical and can carry a lot.

Joe's Rough Guide to Diabetes helps you understand the nature of the disease and how to learn to treat it yourself without ruining your quality of living. Joe's Small-in-one takes this help one step further, giving you the opportunity to treat your diabetes in a way that is as flexible as your lifestyle. I truly believe that with the advice in this booklet and the convenience Joe's Small-in-one affords, you will have all the necessary tools to treat your diabetes effectively and conveniently, and more importantly, to do it Your Way.

Please visit **www.joes-diabetes.com** for further information, or to give feedback on Joe's Rough Guide to Diabetes, or Joe's Small-in-one. All comments are welcome!

[1] "Balance: The guide to testing and treating diabetes", 2009

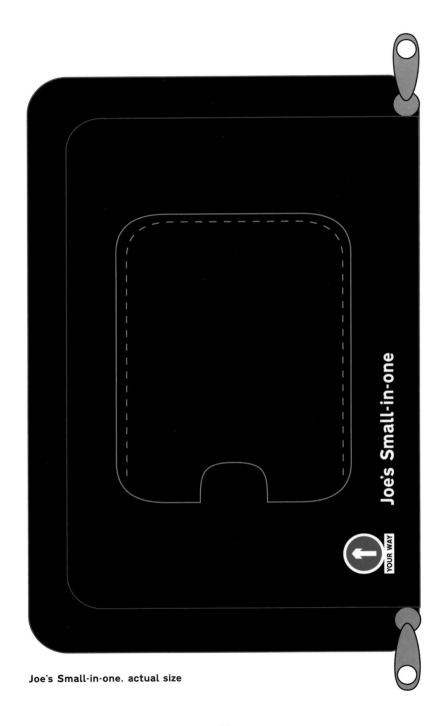

Joe's Small-in-one. actual size

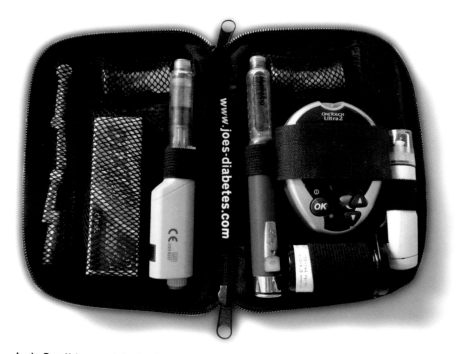

Joe's Small-in-one, interior (not to scale)

10. HELPFUL INFORMATION

High GI foods (GI = 60 to 100)

Food	Portion size	Glycaemic index (GI)	Carbohydrate (g) per portion	kcals per portion
Breakfast cereals				
Cornflakes	1 small bowl (30g)	84	26	108
Rice Crispies	1 small bowl (30g)	82	27	111
Cheerios	1 small bowl (30g)	74	23	111
Shredded Wheat	2 (45g)	67	31	146
Weetabix	2 (40g)	69	30	141
Grains/pasta				
Couscous	5 tbsp (150g)	65	77	341
Brown rice	6 tbsp (180g)	76	58	254
White rice	6 tbsp (180g)	87	56	248
Breads				
Bagel	1 (90g)	72	46	241
Croissant	1 (60g)	67	23	216
Baguette	3 inches long (40g)	95	22	108
White bread	1 large slice (38g)	70	18	85
Wholemeal bread	1 large slice (38g)	69	16	82
Pizza	1 large slice (115g)	60	38	288
Crackers and biscuits				
Puffed crispbread	1 slice (10g)	81	7	32
Ryvita	1 slice (10g)	69	7	32
Water biscuit	1 (8g)	78	6	35
Rice cakes	1 (8g)	85	6	28
Shortbread	1 (13g)	64	8	65
Vegetables				
Parsnip	2 tbsp (65g)	97	8	43
Baked potato	1 medium (180g)	85	22	94
Boiled new potato	7 small (175g)	62	27	116
Mashed potato	4 tbsp (180g)	70	28	188
Chips	average (165g)	75	59	450

Food	Portion size	Glycaemic index (GI)	Carbohydrate (g) per portion	kcals per portion
Swede	2 tbsp (60g)	72	1	7
Broad beans	2 tbsp (120g)	79	7	58
Fruit				
Cantaloupe melon	1 slice (200g)	65	6	26
Pineapple	1 slice (80g)	66	8	33
Raisins	1 tbsp (30g)	64	21	82
Watermelon	1 slice (200g)	72	14	62
Dairy products				
Ice cream	1 scoop (60g)	61	14	62
Drinks				
Fanta	375 ml can	68	51	191
Lucozade	250 ml bottle	95	40	150
Isostar	250 ml can	70	18	68
Gatorade	250 ml bottle	78	15	56
Squash (diluted)	250ml glass	66	14	54
Snacks and sweets				
Tortilla/Corn chips	1 bag (50g)	72	30	230
Mars bar	1 standard (65g)	68	43	287
Muesli bar	1 (33g)	61	20	154
Sugars				
Glucose	1 tsp (5g)	100	5	19
Sucrose	1 tsp (5g)	65	5	19
Maltodextrin	1 tsp (5g)	105	5	19

Moderate GI foods (GI = 40 to 59)

Food	Portion size	Glycaemic index (GI)	Carbohydrate (g) per portion	kcals per portion
Breakfast cereals				
All Bran	1 small bowl (40g)	42	19	104
Sultana Bran	1 small bowl (30g)	52	20	91
Porridge (with water)	1 small bowl (160g)	42	14	78
Muesli	1 small bowl (50g)	56	34	183
Grains/pasta				
Buckwheat	4 tbsp (80g)	54	68	292
Bulgar wheat	4 tbsp (56g)	48	44	196
Basmati rice	4 tbsp (60g)	58	48	215
Noodles	4 tbsp 230g cooked	46	30	143
Macaroni	4 tbsp 230g cooked	45	43	198
Spaghetti	4 tbsp 220g cooked	41	49	229
Breads				
Pitta bread	1 large (75g)	57	43	199
Rye bread	1 slice (25g)	41	11	55
Biscuits and cakes				
Digestive	1 (15g)	59	10	71
Oatmeal	1 (13g)	55	8	57
Rich Tea	1 (10g)	55	8	40
Muffin	1 (68g)	44	34	192
Sponge cake	1 slice (60g)	46	39	181
Vegetables				
Carrots	2 tbsp (60g)	49	3	14
Boiled potato	2 medium (175g)	56	30	126
Peas	2 tbsp (70g)	48	7	48
Sweetcorn	2 tbsp (85g)	55	17	94
Sweet potato	1 medium (130g)	54	27	109
Yam	1 medium (130g)	51	43	173

Food	Portion size	Glycaemic index (GI)	Carbohydrate (g) per portion	kcals per portion
Pulses				
Baked beans	1 small tin (205g)	48	31	166
Fruit				
Apricots	1 (40g)	57	3	12
Banana	1 (100g)	55	23	95
Grapes	1 small bunch (100g)	46	15	57
Kiwi	1 (68g)	52	6	29
Mango	half (75g)	55	11	43
Orange	1 (208g)	44	12	54
Papaya	half (175g)	58	12	47
Peach	1 (121g)	42	8	36
Plum	1 (58g)	39	5	20
Sultanas	1 tbsp (18g)	56	12	50
Dairy products				
Custard	2 tbsp (120g)	43	20	140
Drinks				
Apple juice	1 glass (160ml)	40	16	61
Orange juice	1 glass (160ml)	46	14	58
Snacks and sweets				
Crisps	1 packet (30g)	54	16	159
Milk chocolate	1 bar (54g)	49	31	281
Sugars				
Honey	1 heaped tsp (17g)	58	13	49

Low GI foods (GI = 1 to 39)

Food	Portion size	Glycaemic index (GI)	Carbohydrate (g) per portion	kcals per portion
Breakfast cereals	-	-	-	-
Pulses				
Butter beans	4 tbsp (120g)	31	22	124
Chick peas	4 tbsp (140g)	33	24	168
Red kidney beans	4 tbsp (120g)	27	20	124
Green/brown lentils	4 tbsp (160g)	30	28	164
Red lentils	4 tbsp (160g)	26	28	160
Soya beans	4 tbsp (120g)	18	6	169
Fruit				
Apples	1 (100g)	38	12	47
Dried apricots	5 (40g)	31	15	63
Cherries	1 small handful (100g)	22	10	39
Grapefruit	half (80g)	25	5	24
Peaches tinned	half tin (120g)	30	12	47
Pear	1 (160g)	38	16	64
Plum	1 (55g)	39	5	20
Dairy products				
Full cream milk	half pint (300ml)	27	14	198
Skimmed milk	half pint (300ml)	32	15	99
Yoghurt (low fat fruit)	1 carton (150g)	33	27	135
Snacks and sweets				
Peanuts	1 small handful (50g)	14	4	301
Sugars				
Fructose	1 tsp (5g)	23	5	19

References:
1.Leeds, A, Brand Miller J, Foster-Powell K, Colagiuri S. The Glucose Revolution (2000) (London: Hodder & Stoughton) p29.
2.MAFF/RSC (1991). McCance & Widdowson's The Composition of Foods, 5th ed. (Cambridge: MAFF/RSC)

Useful organisations

Diabetes UK

Macleod House,10 Parkway, London NW1 7AA
Tel: 020 7424 1000 Fax: 020 7424 1001
Email: info@diabetes.org.uk Website: http://www.diabetes.org.uk

This is a useful organisation for all kinds of advice and information about diabetes and also produces the newsletter Balance.

Juvenile Diabetes Research Fund

www.jdrf.org.uk
19 Angel Gate, City Road, London EC1V 2PT
Tel: 020 7713 2030 Fax: 020 7713 2031

Websites

www.diabetes.co.uk
www.diabetes.com
www.diabetes.org (American Diabetes Association)
www.insulin-pumpers.org.uk
www.aventis.com
www.lilly.com
www.abbottdiabetescare.com
www.diabetesnet.com
www.calorieking.com
www.wiki.org
www.nhsdirectwales.nhs.uk
www.joes-diabetes.com
www.talktofrank.com

Handy book

Collins Gem Calorie Counter (available on Amazon.com)

Useful sources of identification bracelets and cards

Medic-Alert Foundation
1 Bridge Wharf, 156 Caledonian Road, London N1 9UU
Tel: 0800 581420 **Email:** info@medicalert.org.uk
Website: http://medicalert.org.uk

Diabetes UK can provide two credit card style identity cards:

Treatment identity card (Order code 7000)
This card has space for you to write in your emergency contact details and where relevant you can record insulin or tablet dosage.
To obtain a treatment identity card, please contact:
Diabetes UK Distribution PO Box 1057, Bedford MK42 7XQ
Tel: 0800 585 088

Insulin user's identity card (Order code 7001)
This card is similar to the card above but also carries your photo and has the phrase 'I have insulin dependent diabetes' in English, French, German, Spanish and Arabic. You can order an insulin user's identity card by completing an application form, available from: **Diabetes UK Customer Services** 10 Parkway, London NW1 7AA **Tel:** 020 7424 1010 **Email:** customerservice@diabetes.org.uk

Blood Ketone Monitoring Advice for people with blood ketone monitors

Ketone reading on your meter (β-OHB (mmol/L))

If your blood glucose is higher than 15mmol/L <u>and you feel unwell</u> you should also measure your blood ketones. The readings on your meter tell you how much β-hydroxybutyrate (β-OHB) is in your blood. If you are in any doubt about your results or your health, contact your local doctor or nurse.

These are acceptable blood ketone levels
Treat your high blood glucose appropriately.

It is important to reduce your blood ketone levels to below 1.0

Take additional short- or rapid-acting insulin. If you do not have this type of insulin use your usual premix insulin. Take 1/5 of your <u>total</u> daily dose. However, if this dose is above 10 units, take just 10 units and contact your healthcare professionals. They may advise you to take more. You should:

- Take insulin

- Retest blood glucose and ketones after 1 hour*

- If your blood glucose and ketones are not falling, contact your doctor or nurse.

- If your blood glucose and ketones are falling, retest every hour while ketones remain above 1.0*

*β-OHB can rise by 1-2 mmol/L per hour. With adequate treatment of diabetic ketoacidosis β-OHB levels should fall by about 1 mmol/L per hour.

Much too high. You are at risk of Diabetic Ketoacidosis (DKA) and the ketone level must be reduced urgently

Take additional short- or rapid-acting insulin. If you do not have this type of insulin use your usual premix insulin. Take 1/5 of your total daily dose, but not more than 10 units. You should:

- Take insulin
- Drink plenty of water
- Seek specialist advice immediately

Please remember to drink at least a cupful of sugar-free fluid every 15mins (about 1 pint or 500mls per hour while your blood glucose is high).

References:
1.The diabetes monitoring forum. www.dmforum.org.uk

It is a good idea to discuss DKA with your diabetes team and make a note of how much insulin they say you should take if you have raised β-OHB. Taking 1/5 of your daily dose is just a guide: it is better to ask what is right for you.

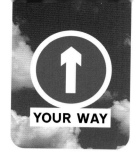

YOUR WAY

Your Way again! You may think it's very boring of me to keep going on about this but, especially when you're newly diagnosed, it's important to get these thoughts clearly in your mind.

Eventually all this diabetes stuff just sinks in and blood sugar regulation becomes almost unconscious, like changing gear in a car. In fact, that's one of my favourite analogies for being diabetic: it's a like moving from an automatic to a manual. The tricky thing is that each person is like a different car, on a different road, in different conditions. Only you, as the driver, know which gear feels right at any moment; or as the diabetic, how much insulin to take.

Experiment safely, and good luck finding Your Way. Happy motoring!

You're responsible
for your diabetes

Only you
can work out how to control your diabetes

Urgent assistance
is required if you have ketoacidosis

Remember to measure
your glucose level before and after you do something new

Whenever you travel
take extra supplies

Always carry
something sweet on you

You have a hidden disability,
but don't let it stop you living your life

NOTES

NOTES

NOTES

NOTES

NOTES

NOTES

NOTES